The Grieving Heart Series:

Depression

Dealing With Depression
Mental Health Support

Aryla Publishing © 2018

www.arylapublishing.com

*Visit the site for more information on books by Fiona Welsh and to be informed of **free promotions!***

Please see other books in my series

The Grieving Heart:-

How To Deal With Financial Stress

The Great Expectations Of Life

Rock That Body: How To Gain Total Body Confidence

Dealing with Death : Finding Your Way After a Loss

Depression: Dealing With Depression Mental Health Support

Anxiety Dealing With Anxiety & Panic Attacks, Mental Health Support

Insomnia : Managing The Stress of Sleep Deprivation

Business & Home Series:-

How to Make Money Online

Keeping Your Children Safe

Contents

Introduction

If you have picked up this book, the chances are that you fall into one of the following categories:

- You are feeling low yourself
- You have been diagnosed with depression
- A loved one has been diagnosed with depression, or is displaying signs of depression
- You are interested in learning more about mental health issues
- You are not sure how you feel, but you are seeking guidance

For any of the situations mentioned above, you have come to the right place. Depression is not something we should sweep under the rug and whisper about, in case someone hears us. It is something to be open and honest about, and something to confront without fear or judgement.

To give you an idea of the sheer size of this problem, Mental Health Foundation estimate that in the past week alone, 1 in 6 adults have experienced a mental health problem of some kind. In addition to this, they also estimate that 7.8% of the UK population alone meet the criteria for diagnosis of depression and anxiety as a mixed condition. This is just in the UK, and it sweeps right across the world too, with NIMH estimating that in 2012, 16 million Americans experienced a form of depression, and the World Health Organisation (WHO) also estimates that on the planet, 350 million people suffer from depression to some degree.

That makes for jaw-dropping reading, right?

This shows you just how prevalent this problem has become, but it also gives you heart that if you are feeling a certain way, you're not alone either. You are not abnormal, there is nothing wrong with you, you are not 'mental', you are simply going through a hard time, and with the right help and support, you will make it out the other side stronger than before. Trust us.

What is Depression?

Depression is such a hard condition to put a label on, because it is invisible, it can't be seen, it can only be felt. If someone tries to explain to you how it feels, you probably won't understand, because it's so different for everyone. On a medical standpoint however, depression is an imbalance in the brain, which affects the way a person thinks, feels, and acts. The episode can be prolonged, it can be short-lived, or it can be intermittent.

Throughout this book we are going to talk in more detail about the symptoms of depression, because that really is the best way to explain what depression actually is. You don't need to get into the medical jargon about the various parts of the brain and why it is all happening, because that won't really help you find any peace. All you need to know is that depression is very real and very common, but it is also very treatable, and there is light at the end of the tunnel. There is nothing wrong with you that cannot be fixed with time and support.

Different Types of Depression

As with anything in life, depression comes in many different forms, and to many different degrees.

Mild depression can be anything from feeling low for a prolonged period of time, to feeling low fleetingly, feeling okay, and then going back to feeling low again. In terms of the medical side of things, there are several recognised types of depression:

- Major depression
- Persistent Depressive Disorder
- Bipolar Disorder

- Seasonal Affective Disorder (SAD)
- Psychotic Depression
- Peripartum/Postpartum Depression
- Premenstrual Dysphoric Disorder
- Situational Depression
- Atypical Depression

All of these are slightly different in their own right, but only because of what actually causes and triggers them. It can be that the symptoms and feelings are the same, but the trigger is different. It could also be that you don't fit into any of the above, and you simply feel very low for no apparent reason – this is still a form of depression.

Now, those medical terms all sound scary, but they are all manageable, treatable, and can be conquered.

What Can You Expect From This Book?

Lots of positivity, lots of helpful information, lots of support, and lots of light at the end of the tunnel! You might be rolling your eyes and thinking this is just another 'think through it' book, but you couldn't be further away from the truth.

The information contained within this book is helpful, practical, and it is designed to help you to see that you are not alone, there is nothing 'mental' about you, and that you can come through this. We totally appreciate that it is going to take hard work and time, but if you are prepared to do that, there is no reason why you can't go back to living a normal, happy, and healthy life.

No-one can judge the way you feel, you own your own feelings, and when you come to terms with that fact, you can start to put into action a slow plan towards recovery. This is what we aim to hep you do. Of course, it might be that it isn't you that is suffering with depression, but a loved one. We will also cover how to deal with this very upsetting and frustrating situation and time in your life, giving you information on what not to do, what to do, and how to look after yourself in the process.

So, without further ado, let's start our journey together.

Chapter 1: The Signs And Symptoms of Depression

Depression is so personal that it is very hard to pinpoint a list of exact signs and symptoms, and to say 'this is what you have when you are depressed'. Everyone feels slightly differently, and they experience symptoms to a different degree. The brain is a very complex and complicated beast, and that means that no diagnosis or symptom chart is ever going to be exact!

Despite that, there are common signs and symptoms to look out for. Of course, the main one is the way you feel in yourself. If you start to feel low for no apparent reason, or if you feel low after a situation in your life but you just can't shake it, you can't get through it, you can't feel hope or happiness, no matter how hard you try; that is the main symptom to look for. There are many physical, emotional, and mental signs and symptoms to look for, and we'll cover those shortly, but it really is mostly about the way you feel in yourself.

This is why depression is so hard to diagnose and pinpoint, because you can't see it. For instance, if you fall over and break your leg, an x-ray can look inside your leg and see the break. The treatment is then super-easy – you get a plaster cast for a few weeks and hopefully it mends quickly and seamlessly. Depression is not like that, because there is no x-ray machine to look inside your brain and see big D floating around, or an imbalance that is visible to the eye. It is all deeply seated in your feelings and outlook, and that's why it is so hard to deal with.

The most difficult part of any depression journey is when it is undiagnosed. Of course, it's hard when you're undergoing treatment, until everything starts to ease and lighten, but in the day when you don't really know what's wrong with you, you feel confused and anxious, scared, and you worry that there is something really wrong with you. It's not until you get a label to put on the way you feel, a term to say 'this is what is happening to me', that you can start to read up on it, understand it, and see that you can cope with it, and that life can get better.

This is why it is so important to recognise and identify the common signs and symptoms of depression. This is especially useful not only for yourself, but for your loved ones too. You can see if someone is displaying any of these signs, and you can keep an eye on that person for any progression. Basically, we all need to know this information, to look after each other.

Physical Signs and Symptoms

Depression isn't just felt on the inside, because a person suffering from depression will, more often than not, display certain physical symptoms too. These are either felt by the person and communicated to others as a complaint, or they are actually visible to others. The most common include:

- Regular headaches – The upset and stress of depression can bring on more headaches when a person is depressed. It is also likely that if you have suffered with migraines in the past, that these will become more intense as you have attacks, and could possibly increase in frequency too
- Back pain – The whole body is under strain when you are depressed, and this can manifest itself in back pain. Again, if you already suffer with back pain regularly, you may notice this becomes worse
- Chronic pain – Anyone who suffers from regular pain, such as joint pain from arthritis, will probably notice that it gets worse during about of depression. Basically, you might feel more aches and pains than normal, and generally feel a little older in terms of your body age
- Chest pain – Now, this is not something to mess around with, so if you do suffer from regular or severe chest pain, do get it checked out by your doctor, but depression can be a cause of chest pain, as well as a fluttering in the

chest, e.g. palpitations. This is quite common when anxiety is mixed in with depression
- A mixture between diarrhoea or constipation – It can be quite common to either alternate between each, or to go in either direction
- Feeling constantly tired no matter how much you sleep - One of the most common signs of depression is feeling and looking constantly tired. This is because even when you sleep, you don't feel totally rested, and you may find it had to get out of bed in the mornings
- General sleep problems – Moving on from our last point, another common physical symptom is sleeping too much, or not sleeping well at all. Again, it can go in either direction but the feeling of tiredness will remain
- Weight and appetite issues – This is anther one which can go in either direction, someone who is depressed can eat too much and put on weight, or not eat at all and lose weight. It is more likely to go in the direction of losing appetite however
- Dizziness and feeling lightheaded – Again, this is most likely experienced when there is an anxiety element to the depression, but overall it is common to feel dizzy for no reason, and a little lightheaded

Remember that everyone is different, so it's possible that you aren't experiencing many of these symptoms, but you're experiencing more of the emotional side of it. It could also be that you only have a few, and not all. These are the most common, it isn't a tick list of having every single one to assure your diagnosis. What this list is mean to do however, is to reassure you that the physical signs and symptoms you are experiencing are normal for someone who is suffering with depression, and nothing to be overly alarmed about per se. Obviously, if they become very troublesome, or you become very worried, then you should definitely seek further medical advice.

Emotional and Mental Signs and Symptoms

The most difficult to discuss symptoms of depression are the ones which are felt, rather then displayed. These are the one which are harder to talk about because they are very difficult to deal with. Not everyone is comfortable taking about their emotions, and explaining how they feel; even the people who are very open can become closed off when suffering from a bout of depression, and it's important to recognise, as with the physical symptoms, that these signs and symptoms go hand in hand with the condition, and not an indicator of anything else.

The most common emotional and mental signs and symptoms of depression are;

- Feel low, to any degree – You might not have a clue why you feel that way, or you might know why but your response to it is more than you would normally feel. You can't seem to shake it, it won't go away, and you can't think of anything else. This is the main emotional and mental symptom of depression, and is the most distressing, whether it is mild or severe
- Feeling hopeless – You can't see a positive in much, and you can't see hope in anything. There is no light at the end of the tunnel for you, you simply feel dark. Many people describe it as feeling like you're drowning, but that everyone else around you is simply fine. You feel jealous and upset that they're okay and you're not feel anything happy at all
- Feeling numb – You might not always feel distressed, you might simply feel nothing at all. Numbness is as much a symptom of depression as feeling everything. Feeling nothing is a dark emotion, and it goes hand in hand with that sense of no hope and also feeling empty
- Feeling anxious a lot of the time – Not everyone suffers from anxiety with depression but the mix of the two is quite common. Anxiety is a whole other set of problems to deal with and when combined it can be very distressing. Feeling worried is one thing, but feeling anxious is something else entirely. Feeling scared ad anxious can lead to feelings of

dizziness, palpitations, and worst case scenarios, and with depression, this can exacerbate completely

- Problems with focus and decision making – You are likely to be unable to concentrate on much for a long period of time, and this is going to make decision making very hard indeed. Work can suffer due to depression, because you simply can't focus on the task at hand, and the lack of sleep combined can make mistakes much more likely
- No energy whatsoever – You're not likely to feel like running a marathon, and you are likely to feel very tired, very easily. Fatigue is one of the most common symptoms of depression
- Feeling very negative – You find it very hard to see a positive, and you become very pessimistic as a result
- Irritability and easy to get angry – The slightest thing can make you angry, and you are likely to be very irritable generally, especially with those you are closest too. This can then lead to feelings of guilt afterwards, because you regret lashing out or saying something you didn't mean
- Lack of wanting to do the things you always used to enjoy – You don't feel the same joy in the things you always used to anymore, and this leads you to closing yourself off to your social circle
- Lack of sex drive – Depression can cause problems in relationships, as a lack of sex drive is one of the most common symptoms
- Possible suicidal thoughts – People with depression can often have thoughts of suicide. It might not mean they are ever seriously gong to consider it, but the thoughts are there. Of course, there is the risk in people with severe depression that suicide could be attempted, so if you do notice suicidal thoughts, this is a red flag to talk to someone you trust.

Again, it's possible to experience just a few or all of these symptoms, but it is the emotional and mental signs and symptoms which are more prevalent than the physical ones.

How Exactly Does it Feel to be Depressed?

Dark, lonely, hopeless, the list goes on. It's very hard to say 'you will feel this way when you are depressed', because as we have mentioned time and time again already, depression is very personal, and everyone feels a slightly different way. Nobody is going to feel full of fairy dust and hope when they are depressed, so from that you can gleam that depression feels very dark and miserable indeed.

If you're not sure whether you are simply feeling a bit under the weather or whether you truly are depressed to some degree, go over those lists of signs and symptoms again and see how many you can tick off. If you are agreeing with several of them, it is a good indicator that you should head to see your doctor and have a chat.

Now we know how it feels, what to look for, and the signs and symptoms of depression, we need to give some consideration to what actually causes it.

Chapter 2: Causes of Depression

What causes depression? Well, the list can be as long as your arm!

We know that depression in its most medical form is caused by a chemical imbalance in the brain, and that chemical change can be down to several factors, including hormones, genetics, different medical conditions, as well as stressful situations in life.

These days, we live such busy lives that we are constantly on the go, and we are feeling pressured to do everything, ticking everything off our list. This isn't always possible, and the disappointment can lead to feelings of worthlessness. In certain situations, that feeling can then send you down a further spiral, and before you know it, you're within the depression bracket.

Causes and triggers are different things, so we need to really highlight to slight change between them there. Triggers are personal, they are situations or things which are personal to you, and which can trigger a sense of feeling down, or of a depressive bout, within you as an individual. Causes are more widespread and universal, these are things which are known to contribute to the development of depression amongst most people. Just because you have experienced one of the situations on the cause list doesn't mean you are bound to become depressed, but it can make it more likely.

Common Causes of Depression

Hormones
Whilst hormonal changes are much more likely to affect women than men, it's not unheard of for a hormonal cause to be the reason by a male depression. For now however, let's focus on the women, because this category is much more adherent to the females out there.

Basically, there are three main times in life when hormones could play a part in depression – menstruation (periods), childbirth, and the menopause. These are all milestones in a woman's life and they have a habit of throwing hormones out of whack. Of course, that doesn't mean that there aren't other times in life when hormonal imbalances occur, and this in itself can be a cause for depression.

This is all down to the fact that hormones are chemicals, and we know that depression is caused by a chemical imbalance. When your hormones aren't working at the right levels, it can cause you to feel low, out of sots, and it can develop into depression. We know that postpartum depression (or more commonly known as postnatal depression) is something we're all warned about when we become pregnant and have children. This is because your body goes through so many changes during pregnancy and childbirth, that it really does send your hormones all over the place. This can cause an imbalance and it can cause depression. Similarly, when you enter and go through the menopause, again, hormones are not always within the right ranges, as they should be. Again, during menstruation, some women experience period problems, which is down to an issue with their hormonal levels.

When you go to your doctor and talk about the way you're feeling, it's likely that they might take a blood test for hormone levels, especially if you are of menopausal age, you've just had a baby, or you complain of period issues. If this comes back showing that your hormone levels are deranged, then medication, e.g. hormonal manipulation, could be an option to look into.

Genetics
Now, genetics do play a part in whether you are more likely to develop depression or not. If you have several family members who have suffered from moderate to severe depression then your chances of developing depression are a little higher too.

Of course, this doesn't mean you are definitely going to develop the condition, but it means you have more chance. On the flip side however, you could be the first within your family to develop it, and that could be because your cause is something else entirely, e.g. a situation that has occurred in your life, a medical condition, or a hormonal problem.

If you do have several family members who have had depression then it is just a warning sign to be a little more aware of how you feel. If you notice yourself becoming down and having thoughts that are aligned with a depressive state then it's a good idea to seek out help a little sooner, as the chances of you going down that dark path are a little higher.

The reason that genetics are part of the causes is that again, it's down to chemicals. DNA and all that jazz runs around the body, makes us what we are and basically does a lot of very complicated work in the body and the brain. We know that a chemical imbalance is the medical cause of depression, so it makes sense that genetics could play a part somewhere in the jigsaw puzzle.

Certain Medical Conditions
There are some medical conditions which can make the sufferer a little more predisposed to developing depression and a lot of this is down to the medication that person takes to treat the medical condition they have. Again, if depression is a side effect of a medication you are taking, that doesn't mean you are definitely going to develop it, it just means that it is a possibility and you should be aware and monitor the way you are feeling.

The most common medical conditions that have a link with depression development are;
- Lupus
- Diabetes
- Heart Disease
- Hypothyroidism
- Arthritis

- Kidney disease
- Multiple Sclerosis (MS)
- HIV/AIDS

Again, it's about being aware of the possible risk, not a definite sentence towards depression.

Situations in Life
Without a doubt, one of the most common causes of becoming depressed is that something has happened in your life and it has caused the depression, due to the way you think after the event, feelings of hurt, confusion, negativity, etc. Common situations include the loss of a job, the loss of someone we love, a relationship break up, cheating, money problems, or someone close to us becoming ill. It doesn't have to be something massive either, it can be something small, or it can be a snowball effect of bad luck or situations that cumulate in you feeling down over a long period of time.

Of course, it could also be that you simply don't know why you're feeling down, but there is likely to be something that has happened to trigger it. Again, we'll talk about triggers in a later section, as this is something a little more personal overall.

We Can't do it All!

Another cause, something which doesn't really fit any of the moulds above, but something which has become prevalent in our busy lives these days, is social pressures. For instance, social media – the comparisons that are made from social media can dent a person's confidence down to the point where they become very low indeed. We are going to talk in a later chapter about the role of social media, because it is so important to highlight.

For now however, we'll talk about the pressure of having to do it all. We are supposed to be a mother or a father, a husband or a wife, a boyfriend or a girlfriend, a son or a daughter, a good friend, a great employee, a great boss, we're supposed to run the house seamlessly, we're not supposed to forget to pay our bills, we have to make ends meet, we can't forget to do anything, and we have to do all of this with a big smile on our face and not complain.

How is anyone supposed to cope with this situation for a long period of time without becoming down at least once or twice? The problem is when that prolonged pressure becomes too much and it knocks a person down to the point where depression sets in. We cannot do it all, it is impossible. We compare ourselves to the man or woman down the street who seems to have all their life in order, and we start to feel bad about ourselves. The problem is, we only see the outside; that man or woman probably cries themselves to sleep at night because they're so stressed out.

Our busy lives and social pressures certainly have an impact on the way we feel, and this is one of the modern day's biggest causes of depression amongst adults.

Know Your Personal Triggers

So, we've talked about the causes of depression, and we've talked about why they are causes, but we need to talk abut personal triggers now, as we become more personal in our approach.

As we mentioned, causes are mainstream, triggers are personal. What are your triggers? How do you identify them?

The thing is, if you can identify your triggers then you ca put mechanisms into place to avoid them, and then you can keep an even keel on your emotions and hopefully avoid depressive bouts from occurring, or minimising them as much as possible.

Do you become very down at work? If so, this could be a sign that you need to think about changing your job. In that case, your work is your trigger.

Do you become down when you start to think about a situation in your past that is unresolved? In that case, the memories of that issue are your trigger. The way to deal with them is to either seek counselling to gain closure, or find a way to become more at peace with the issue.

Does a certain place cause you to sink into depression at certain memories from your childhood, perhaps? In that case, the place is your trigger. Can you avoid it? If so, that's your answer.

As you can see, identifying your trigger is about thinking about how certain things make you feel, ad how your thoughts go on from there. You only have to really consider the way something makes you feel in your gut, and your physical and emotional reactions to it, to find out whether that particular thing, memory, or person is your actual trigger.

Some serious soul searching needs to be done here, and it might not even be a physical thing, it could be a memory, or a thought; the point however is, once you know what that trigger is, you can either avoid it altogether, manage it, or conquer it, depending on which is the best course of action for you.

Your Emotional Checklist

So far we have covered a lot of ground, and we have thrown a lot of information at you. You picked up this book because you have an interest in learning more about depression, and hopefully because you want to help yourself too. In order to find out whether you actually are depressed, or whether you think you could be going that way, you need to really think about how you feel. Now, this might not be an easy task for you, and it might be unpleasant, but we have to do such things in order to be able to conquer our greatest fears.

Every morning when you wake up, you need to do a quick emotional checklist, a health MOT of sort.

- How do you feel?
- Did you sleep well?
- Are you fearful of anything that is going to happen that day?
- Do you feel hopeful for the day, or do you feel worried?

Monitor this over a few days.

At the end of each day, before you sleep, ask yourself the following questions.

- How do you feel now, at the end of the day?
- Are you very tired, or just normally tired?
- How do you feel about the way the day went?
- Do you think the day went well?
- What problems did you encounter, and can you put them to rest before the next day starts?

The point of asking yourself these questions is that you will give yourself an overview of how you feel over a segment of time. It's normal for us to feel a bit 'bleurgh' from day to day, this is totally fine, but when you feel that way over along period of time, and you don't answer 'yes' so whether you feel hopeful or not, you are giving yourself important information that perhaps you need to seek out a little help and support, before the problem becomes worse.

You could even write these answers down in a notebook, to give you a mood diary of sorts, and this will help you to see if there are any areas you could work on, or any areas of concern.

Chapter 3: Depression Diagnosis & Treatment

The bravest thing you can do as an adult human being is to say 'help me'. There is no weakness, no failures, and no faults in doing this, it is the strongest and the most brave thing you can ever do and say.

As adults we are told that we have to be strong, we have to keep a stiff upper lip, keep calm and carry on, but that is actually totally against what we should be doing. Yes, we need to be strong in situations and we should just keep calm and get on with it most of the time, but when we are struggling, when we need help, we shouldn't brush it under the carpet and hope it goes away, perhaps giving it the chance to get worse, we need to reach out.

There is so much help out there for anyone who is struggling with low mood and depression of any type or degree, and the first step towards recovery is a simple reach out towards that helping hand. It is the hardest step, that's for sure, but it is the most brave and most rewarding one you will travel in your life.

The thing is, once we reach out, we can get help, we can start our journey to recovery, and that shining light at the end of the tunnel becomes a full on laser beam.

Where to Get Help

The most common place to head is to see your doctor. If you don't want to see your family doctor, you can ask to see another doctor in the practice, safe in the knowledge that everything you say in that room is totally confidential, and will not be communicated to anyone else. Your GP is expertly trained in dealing with depression, because it has become so prevalent. You are not the first person to walk through those doors and talk about how they feel, and you certainly will not be the last.

If you don't want to see your GP, there are other places you can go, such as private practices, but to be honest, it is much better to see your doctor. Your local doctor has the records of your overall health from birth, and if there is a problem with depression, this should be on your record too. Remember, everything is private, nothing is judged, and your GP can help you manage your condition at a local level.

Of course, prior to this, if you want to speak to someone, there are many helplines you can call, such as Samaritans. We're going to list some of the helpful organisations you can contact at he end of the book, but these organisations are there to offer a helping hand and a listening ear to anyone who is struggling. Sometimes, simply having someone listen to the way you feel can make you feel like a weight has been lifted, and a lot of the time people feel better when it is someone they don't know. Local support groups can also help, because being around people who feel the same way as you can often be a real lift.

As you can see, there is a lot of help out there, as well as a lot of online groups and resources to access too. You are never alone, even though you may feel that way at first

How is Depression Diagnosed?

In order for depression treatment to start, you first need to visit a doctor and have a chat. You will sit down with him or her and you'll just tell them how you feel. This sounds so simple in practice, but we totally understand that it can be a difficult thing to do in reality. Remember, nothing goes outside of the walls you are within, you are safe, and you are respected, you are not judged, and you are listened too completely.

The doctor will then listen to you and ask you some questions. You will be asked about your appetite, how you're sleeping, whether you're eating, you'll probably be asked about your thoughts, e.g. whether you have had any suicidal thoughts, but this is something that they have to ask, in order to ascertain the level to which you are feeling.

Whilst you are with the doctor, they will write notes, so don't be alarmed by this, it is just help them write down and note what you are saying. It might also be the case that you are asked to give a blood test, to help rule out any hormonal imbalance causes, the types we were talking about earlier.

After taking a full medical history, talking to you about how you are feeling, and sometimes a medical examination, your doctor will be able to diagnose you with depression, or otherwise. There are no specific tests to say 'yes' you have it, or 'no' you don't, which is what makes the whole shebang so mysterious and difficult. Your doctor however knows what to look for.

Common Treatment Options

Before we start talking about how to treat depression, we need to point out one thing – every single person is different, we are all individual, and that means that one size doesn't always fit all. Depression treatment is often a trial and error kind of deal, because your doctor needs to find out the route and the combination of medication or otherwise which you respond to as an individual. Just because Jane down the road is on a certain medication once per day and is feeling wonderful, doesn't mean that particular medication is going to work for you! It might not even be about medication for you, there are other options for treatment.

The main and most common treatment options are:

- Antidepressant medications
- Cognitive Behavioural Therapy (CBT)
- Counselling

There are some alternative methods, but these aren't generally approved and recognised as being official lines of treatment, so we will stick to the ones which are.

Now, the words 'antidepressant medications' can be worrying, but these medications are given in different dosages, and have varying degrees of side effects. Again, it will b a slow process to find out which one works for you, and they don't work overnight, but once the medication builds up in your system, and it begins to work, you will start to feel better. After that, your doctor will decide how long to keep you on the medication, and whether to keep you on a low maintenance dose, or whether to slowly wean you off them over time. This will be a decision you will make together, and after discussion about how you are feeling.

Cognitive Behavioural Therapy, more commonly known as CBT, is about learning to change the way you think, to avoid the triggers that cause your depressive symptoms, and to help you learn lifelong managing techniques. This is often offered in conjunction with medications, and has been proven to be very effective. Of course, not everyone responds to CBT, and that can sometimes be because certain people can find it hard to open up. If you give it at try fully however, and really open yourself up to the process, you will find that it is very beneficial indeed.

Finally on our list we have counselling. If there is a situation in your life or in your past which is your trigger, something you are struggling to deal with, and something which is contributing to the way you feel, then counselling can hep you. Again, it's about coping mechanisms and thinking about how to change the way you feel and think about a situation, but it can be very useful in order to get closure on a painful or troublesome situation in your life. Many people think that counselling is like the therapy sessions you see on TV, but it is actually a much more interactive and involved method these days, and doesn't usually involve lying on a couch!

Of course, there are ways that you can help yourself a little too, and in our next chapter we are going to explore them in a little more detail. If you work these self-help methods alongside your formal treatment for depression, you will find that your response is much faster as a result.

Chapter 4: How to Help Yourself

We have covered the medical and cognitive ways that depression is treated, but we now need to talk about the ways that you can help yourself in your recovery and management of depression.

There are actually a lot of things that you can do to help make yourself feel better. but the difficulty comes when you simply don't feel motivated to even get out of bed, let alone go and do some exercise. Once you begin your route towards recovery, you need to push yourself to at least try. You have done the hardest thing by admitting that you need help, by starting your medication, and by speaking to your doctor, and now you need to push a little further and exert some of that will to feel better.

You can find it within yourself if you dig deep enough, and whilst it is going to feel like a mammoth effort at the start, keep in your mind as much as possible that if you do this, you are going to feel better, you are going to start to feel lighter, and you are going to see a sunny day and feel good about it as a result.

Most of self-help is about being compliant with your medication, attending your counselling sessions and giving CBT a try, but it's also about embracing good health and well-being, and it's about pushing yourself to get out of your comfort zone. Again, at first it wont be easy, but challenge yourself to at least try, give it a month, and see how you feel – the results will see you wanting to carry on.

Lifestyle Changes

By lifestyle changes we mean taking a long hard look at your diet, your exercise regime and how much sleep you are getting. The chances that you aren't exercising much and that your eating habits have gone totally out of whack, thanks to the effects of your depression. This needs to change, and these small changes can turn into a huge snowball effect over a short space of time.

The following are lifestyle changes you can make that will make a massive difference;

- **Eat properly** – Embrace healthy and clean eating. This will not only cleanse your body of any impurities and toxins, but it will give you more of a spring in your step. Avoid processed, fried foods, and make sure you load up your diet with fresh fruit and vegetables, lean meats, fish, plenty of water, and that you get your 5 a day as much as possible.

- **Get enough sleep** – At first this is going to be difficult, especially if you are finding it hard to sleep as part of your depression. Try relaxation techniques before bed, such as meditating, or turning off the TV and reading a book instead, drink a warm, milky drink, and listen to gentle, calming music. The easier you find it to nod off, the more sleep you will get, and when you get into a regular pattern of 6-8 hours every night, your body will start to feel rejuvenated. Avoid oversleeping, and make yourself get out of bed in the mornings, push yourself to do it, because too much sleep can be just as bad as not enough.

- **Relax and switch off** – It's important to have 'me' time every single day, even if it's just an hour. Do something you used to enjoy, and try and recapture that enjoyment. If not, try and find something new and develop that into a hobby. Perhaps join a night class and learn a new skill, and you'll find this not only relaxes your frazzled mind, but it helps to boost your confidence in yourself too.

- **Exercise** – One of the biggest natural mood boosters out there is exercise. Get outside if you can and go for a walk or a run, the fresh air, nature, and the fact you're exercising will help to get your blood pumping, help clear your head, and get your body moving. The endorphins will start to be released, and you'll feel lighter over time, even if it doesn't feel that way at first. It doesn't have to be the gym you join, but if you want to, go for it! Try a team sport, join an exercise class, play tennis, or basically just go for a walk every day.

- **Be sociable** – This is probably going to be the hardest one of them all, because when you are feeling depressed, you do not want to socialise, you want to hibernate. The thing is, when you hibernate you are feeding that depressive seed and allowing it to grow. If you can find it in yourself to push yourself out of the house and out for a coffee or a tea with a friend, you will feel better by the end of it, and you will slowly find it easier to do over time. It doesn't have to be something huge or expensive, it can simply be a walk around the park with the dogs, incorporating some exercise, or it can be a quick hour for lunch somewhere. Basically just try and get back some of your old social life. We mentioned that evening class idea a little earlier, and that is a great way to meet new people too.

- **Avoid drinking, smoking, and alcohol** – These are three big triggers and exacerbations for depression and should be avoided. Unhealthy coping mechanisms only give you a very temporary high, before dropping you down further than you were before. Kick them out of your life and stick to the healthy highs, such as exercise and new hobbies instead. No-one is saying that you can never have a glass of wine or a beer ever again, but whilst you are recovering from your depression, this is something you need to avoid for now, and afterwards, only in moderation.

Turning Negatives Into Positives

There is a very handy CBT trick that you can learn and do on your own. When you are in a depressed state, you are not feeling very positive, and everything is rather dark and negative. The thing is, negativity breeds negativity, and that breeds depression. What you need to try and do is turn those negative thoughts into positives ones, and then allow them to bloom over time.

This isn't going to happen overnight, and it will take a fair bit of effort at first, but the hope is that over time it will become second nature to think this way, rather than the old way.

- Be aware of your thoughts. The next time you have a negative thought, allow it to flow into your mind.
- Now, firmly say in your mind (not aloud unless you want strange looks), 'No!' and visualise yourself pushing that thought away with your hand.
- Now, you need to think of a positive thought to replace that negative one. So for example, if your thought was 'why does it always rain', think 'I'm going to buy myself a new umbrella', and make good on your promise.
- The next time that thought comes into your head, repeat it, so when it rains, remember that new umbrella you bought, in a bright colour.
- Over time, the hope is that your brain will begin to remember the positive rather than the negative, but repetition is key, so you need to keep reminding your brain of the good things about rain, for example.

It might seem like a waste of time, but it really does work. It takes time and effort, but it does work to replace old mind-sets with new ones. If that rain analogy doesn't work for you, it could be a negative thought like 'Mavis at work is really annoying', and you could then change it and say 'Mavis at work is good at her job'. You then repeat it over and over again, and hopefully Mavis will cease to become quite so annoying to you!

Dealing With Setbacks

We need to give a quick mention to the possibility of setbacks along your recovery journey. These are possible, and whilst we hope they don't happen to you, we do need to arm you with the right information to help you get through it unscathed.

Basically, when you are on the road to recovery, that nasty little depression in your head doesn't want you to win. It will do whatever it can to drag you back down, a little like a devil on your shoulder. It could also be a situation which has occurred fresh in your life. Basically, do not let that little devil win, and do not let that situation set you back. If you feel like you need extra help, head back to your doctor and explain how you feel, it may be that your medication needs adjusting a little. You could also make an appointment with your counsellor to talk through it all. The key however is that you recognise the setback, ad you don't allow it to become a major issue in your already fantastic recovery.

Chapter 5: Common Misconceptions Around Mental Health

This chapter is about smashing myths and misconceptions and allowing you to see the truth about depression and its prevalence in today's society. We talked in our introduction section about a few statistics an we talked about how common depression is, but to feel totally at ease with your situation, you need to understand that you are not alone, and you are actually in very good company indeed.

People don't like to talk about mental health issues, but that is what depression is a part of. Mental health isn't about being in a straightjacket or being crazy, it's about dealing with life's ups and downs in the best way we can, and admitting that occasionally we need a bit of help to cope. Almost every single person on the planet has experienced a mental health problem to some degree at some point in their lives, even if it's just a short period of low mood. It's time we learnt to be more open and honest about our mental health, to shatter that illusion that there is something taboo, or strange about it.

Depression, mental health, any type of issue which involves the mind is so common, so ridiculously common, that to have any type of worry abut talking about it and admitting that you feel a certain way is actually crazy in itself. These days more and more celebrities are speaking out about their own mental health issues, and this is a great thing, because it helps youngsters in particular to see that to feel a certain way and to struggle occasionally isn't something to be ashamed of – if their hero is admitting to it then they don't feel quite so bad about it too.

Even the Royal Family are getting in on the act, with Princes William and Harry, as well as Kate Middleton, heading up a charity to bring to attention mental health, whilst talking bout their own experiences after the death of their mother. Again, this is a hugely positive step towards smashing the taboos that unfortunately still exist today when it comes to mental health problems and issues in society and beyond.

Men & Depression – Get Rid of The Taboo

Whether we want to admit it or not, men these days are expected to still be MEN. They are exacted to cope with everything, they are expected to provide, and they are not expected to talk about their feelings and their emotions. This needs to change.

Men are human beings, they have ups and downs in life just like the rest of us, they have feelings, they have emotions, they cry, they feel sad, they feel happy. Whether you admit it or not, men are just not supposed to feel upset or emotional.

Wrong!

This taboo of depression and mental health issues and men has to stop, because it is so hugely damaging. This is stopping men from reaching out and getting help for the way they feel, and that is why so many men these days simply don't go to the doctor, and allow it to develop too far. The frightening thing is that according to Mental Health Foundation, suicide is the mot common cause of death in men aged between 20 and 49 years in the UK. Can you imagine how many of those men could have been saved if they'd felt they could go and talk to someone? If they didn't feel like they just weren't supposed to cry, and that they were less of a man for admitting they were upset?

It has to stop now!

Humans are humans, whether male, female, or gender neutral – we all cry, we all feel fear, anger, upset, sadness, happiness, joy, jealousy, and everything above and beyond that. Depression is something we have to deal with in our lives these days, and whilst we all wish that wasn't the case, the fact that people feel that a man is less of a man for admitting he needed help is quite frankly ridiculous! As we mentioned, the strongest thing you can do as a human, the strongest thing you can do as a man, is to say 'I need help'.

The Potential Role of Social Media

There is a debatable role of social media in terms of the rise of depression prevalence in today's society, and that really comes down to comparisons and confidence levels.

Instagram and Facebook are packed with photos of people filtered to look their very best, full of amazing holiday snaps, and status updates about how much they love their man/girlfriend, and how lucky they are, blah blah. The thing is, half the time it isn't true, and said person is only posting this to make themselves feel better. As humans, some of us somehow feel that dragging someone else down, builds us up. If you are feeling a little low in the first place, subjecting yourself to this can actually make you feel ten times worse.

You might not even realise it is happening, but if you are noticing your mood becoming al little lower, it could be a good idea to give yourself a social media break. Log out of your accounts for a week and see how you feel. This is something which is becoming more and more common amongst especially the 20-40 year age group.

A Few Useful Statistics

To further drive home the size of the depression problem on the globe, let's talk stats. Some of these have already been mentioned, but let's keep them all in one handy place, for future reference.

- It is estimated that 1 in 6 people in the past one week along have experienced a mental health problem to some degree – Mental Health Foundation

- It is estimated that a huge 7.6% of the UK population actually meet the criteria for diagnosis of depression and anxiety combined – Mental Health Foundation
- 1 in 6 adults have suffered from a mental health problem in the UK alone – Mental Health Foundation
- It is estimated that a combined anxiety and depression condition contributes to 1/5 of all days off sick from work – Mental Health Foundation
- In the UK, suicide is the most common cause of death amongst men aged between 20-49 years – Mental Health Foundation
- At any given time, 10% of mothers, and 6% of men are suffering from mental health problems in the UK – Mental Health Foundation
- Women are more likely to be diagnosed with a mental health problem in the UK than men, and twice as likely to be diagnosed with an anxiety disorder – Mental Health Foundation
- It is estimated that 350 million people across the globe are suffering from depression – World Health Organisation (WHO)

Eye opening stuff, you'll probably agree.

Chapter 6: When It's Not You – How to Cope When a Loved One is Suffering From Depression

When someone close to you is suffering from any form of depression, it can be a very lonely, upsetting, and frustrating time. You may find that you are the source of their irritation, that you are the one they lash out to, and that you are the one they shut out the most.

How to deal with this is very difficult, but it is so vital not to take it personally. This might sound ridiculously impossible, because if someone you love more than anything else in the world is shutting you out and becoming irritated at you for no reason of course it's going to hurt you, but you need to remember that this isn't the real them acting out. They are venting their frustration at the way they are feeling inside, and they do not mean what they are saying. Of course, nobody expects you to just stand there and take it, soak it all up like a sponge and let it bounce off you, but at the same time, becoming embroiled in a fight or argument is not going to help at all either.

You need to be superman or superwoman in this case, and as hard as it is going to be, you need to be strong for the both of you.

Let's try and navigate this very difficult situation.

What is the Right Approach?

There are certain things you should never say to someone who is obviously suffering with depression, whether they are diagnosed or not. Never tell them to 'get over it', and never tell them to 'smile'. Put yourself in their shoes for a minute – do you think they want to feel this way? Of course not. Now, we're not suggesting that you are in any way that insensitive, but when you are so frustrated with someone, so concerned, and so hurt at the way things are playing out, it's so easy to just say something insensitive off the cuff. Try and bite your tongue as much as possible – you will get your rewards, honestly!

The first thing to think about is whether or not your loved one is getting help or not. If they have made that step towards recovery and reached out to their doctor then that's great, and you need to continue to be supportive in their journey, taking each day as it comes, and not thinking ahead too much. There are going to be setbacks occasionally, so simply be aware of it and deal with them as they arise. Make sure your loved ones takes their medication, but don't become too motherly about it, don't remind them abut it on the hour, every hour – simply carefully check that they are taking it as they should.

Try and encourage them gently to get out of the house, perhaps suggesting going out for a walk, or a run, or maybe even heading out for lunch. If they refuse, don't become upset or take it personally, just try again a few days later. Also be aware that they might start spending time with a friend, rather than you. Again, this is going to be hurtful, but if it gets them out of the house, try and see it as a positive. Some people, especially men, find it easier to communicate their feelings to someone they aren't so close to, and if you are their partner, their mother, their sister etc, you might not be the person they choose to spill all too. If you are, that's great, but if not, just try and be happy that they are talking it out to someone, and that they are getting out of the house, provided it's not all the time.

Try and cook healthy meals, incorporate fresh fruit and vegetables as much as possible, and keep alcohol out of the house too. Try and take the pressure off a little, so if your partner is always the one doing the house work, help out a little, and if they are always fetching the kids from school, you do it a couple of times a week instead. Basically, just let them recover gently, whilst still keeping their sense of independence and need too.

If your partner is not diagnosed, then your job is to try and gently encourage them to get help. You might be met with a barrage of abuse at some point, but again, let it bounce off you. Admitting you need help is the hardest part. Leave a few leaflets lying around the house strategically, drop a few hints into conversations. Of course, it does pay to sit down and try and talk to your loved one and get them to go and get help too, but this has to be their decision ultimately, so go gently wherever possible.

Keep an Eye on Your Own Mental Health

There is a lot of debate over which situation is easier, it is easier to be the person dealing with the depression, or the person dealing with the person with the depression? Who knows, only you both know how you feel inside, but it's definitely a hard situation to be the one watching a loved one suffer so much. You are going to feel pushed out, as we mentioned, and you're going to feel lonely, but it's vital to remember that this is not going to last forever, that there will be better days again, and you'll come out of this stronger together, no matter what capacity your relationship or friendship is.

One thing to note however is that you need to keep an eye on the way you feel too. It's very easy for you to become depressed in this situation too, because you're surrounded by it, and you're bound to feel a little low yourself. You're not made of steel, it's going to hurt you, so you need to keep an eye on your own mental health. Remember to incorporate the self help techniques we were taking about easier into your own routine, and to seek help immediately if you start to feel like you could be going down the same road as your loved one.

Chapter 7: Helpful Websites & Organisations

Anxiety UK
www.anxietyuk.org.uk

Bipolar UK
www.bipolaruk.org.uk

CALM – The Campaign Against Living Miserably (for men aged between 15-35)
www.thecalmzone.net

Depression Alliance – A full network of groups for self-help
www.depressionalliance.org

Mental Health Foundation
www.mentalhealth.org.uk

MIND
www.mind.org.uk

Rethink Mental Illness
www.rethink.org

Samaritans
www.samaritans.org.uk

SANE
www.sane.org.uk/support

Conclusion

We hope that this book has been helpful to you, and that you are now feeling a lot more proactive about conquering your depression once and for all. Remember that you are not alone in this journey towards a more positive state of mind, and that there is always help and support out there.

Never feel like you are different, wrong, strange, or anything else negative for being depressed. We have highlighted so many times about how prevalent depression is in today's society, and that means that you probably met countless people in your life who have suffered with depression too – they might have been suffering with it at the time of your meeting, but they were hiding it really well.

If there is any part of this book that you feel you need to go back over again, go for it. This book is there as a reference point and a confidence booster whenever you feel you need it. Also, if you feel there is anyone in your life who could benefit from our help, let them have a read too – we want to help as many people as possible.

There are so many misconceptions and myths about mental health that need shattering. We need to be able to speak out and be honest about our feelings and our emotions, and about our problems.

We wish you luck on your journey, whatever point you are at, and hope that the information contained within this book has helped you in some way.

Thank you for reading my book.

I would love it if you could leave me an honest review on what you thought of this book.

If you like to know more about my books and the opportunity to be notified of free promotions please visit Aryla Publishing website

Or follow Facebook, Instagram and Twitter @arylapublishing

Thank you

Please see other Titles from

ARYLA PUBLISHING Visit

www.arylapublishing.com

to sign up for new release books and free promotions

Children's Books

The Body Goo Series

The Billy Series

Adult Books

Self Help Books

Diet and Wellbeing

Comedy Books

Other Publications

How to be a World Leader – By Tyler Moses
(Comedy)

The year is 2017 and while none of us know what the future will hold at present we are at the mercy of a world leader in the USA that did not seem possible. But it has happened some ask how? Some ask why? But there is support out there so I say if he can do it then so can I and so can you!

If you are not automatically born into it and lucky enough to be an heir to a kingdom (we will also cover how to bump yourself up the ranks) if you have the unfortunate sibling line to contend with that does not put you in prime position.

In the world, we live in today with technology at our fingertips we have more control and access to information so make use of it the world is your oyster if you have visions of being the most powerful person in the world and have an unstoppable ego then this could be the job for you.

Keeping Your Children Safe – By Fiona Welsh (Self Help – Business)

Without a doubt, the most important and treasured things we have in our lives are our children. We give birth to them, we raise them, we worry about them, and we love them to the end of the world and back again. It is no surprise that when we see worrying events on the news, it first makes us think of our children.

We can't protect our kids from everything in life, and we can't shield them from the things that are going on around the globe, but we can do our very best to keep them as safe as possible. As a parent you will no doubt be very familiar with the thought that you want to wrap your children up in cotton wool and avert their eyes from anything that isn't Disney magical. Things can and do happen, but part of the solution is to know how to teach your children about safety in general, in the right way. Learning to show them that it is fine to explore, fine to live, but that being on the lookout for danger is vital.

So, how do you do that? How do you tread that fine line between living life and avoiding dangerous situations?

How to Make Money Online –
By Fiona Welsh (Self Help – Business)

Unfortunately, the pot of gold at the end of the rainbow is yet to be found, there doesn't seem to be a Leprechaun smiling at whoever manages to stumble upon this long-famed prize, and as for the money tree, well, it's still as elusive as ever.

From time to time, we all find money hard to come by, and no matter how hard we work, or how much we save, it's likely that there are things we want and need that we can't afford at the present time. Obviously, that doesn't mean that your money situation is going to be difficult all the time, because cash flow ebbs and flows (pardon the pun) as much as anything in life, but finding ways to help it along a little is always a good thing.

The internet has changed so much about our modern-day lives, it is quite hard to think of anything that we don't use an online connection for in some way or another. From booking holidays, doing our grocery shopping, meeting the new Mr or Mrs Right in our lives, or finding a new job, the Internet connects it all. So, taking that thought a little further, can the Internet help us to earn a little extra cash when our flow isn't, well, flowing as fast as we would like?

Of course, it can!

The Internet is a fantastic place to start, and the beauty of all of it is that you can do it from the comfort of your armchair!

Julia's Dilemma – By Lyndsey Carter (Romantic Comedy)

Julia sighed as she stepped onto the escalator. As it moved and took her up, she sighed again. Another boring day and another crammed ride home on a smelly train with no seats. She longed for some excitement, something to shake things up. She was sick of the same old, same old.

Julie boarded the train, already knowing as she craned her neck to scan each corner that there would not be any seats open. Instead, she settled for a hand-hold on the pole near the back wall. But her surroundings ceased to bother her as she stared off into the distance and let her thoughts roam. She looked at the houses she passed and imagined what type of people lived there. The train line ran at the back of the houses giving Julie a view of the garden. Some gardens had washing hanging up; others had kids' toys. Some gardens were overgrown like a mini jungle. It was a little daydream game Julie liked to play when she didn't have a book or paper to read. Soon the passing gardens and motion of the train made her eyes heavy.

Julia fought to keep her eyes open, scared that she would miss her stop. Even after six years of riding the same train back and forth to work, she was still afraid that she would fall asleep and ride until the train reached the end of the line.

The mechanical voice announced the train's next stop, and that was enough to wake Julia.

We also have a selection of Adult Coloring Books to help relax pass the time and de-stress.

Beautiful Illustrations and puzzles in the back for your entertainment.

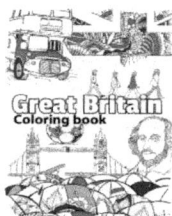

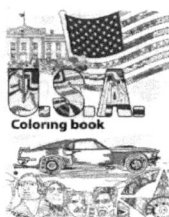

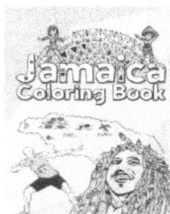

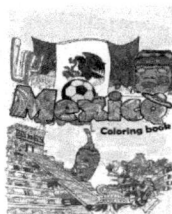

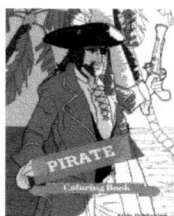

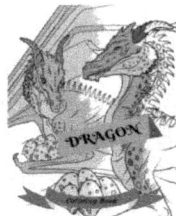

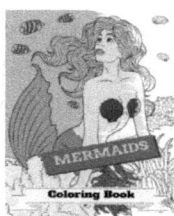

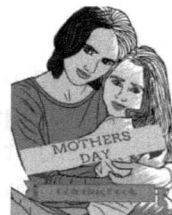

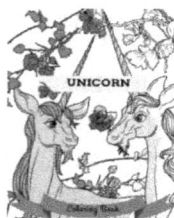

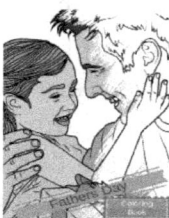

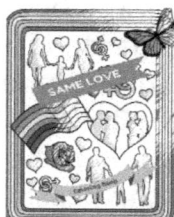

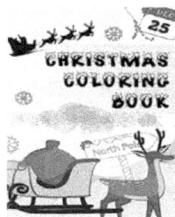

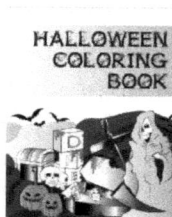

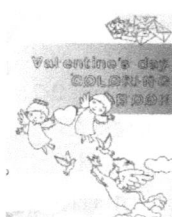

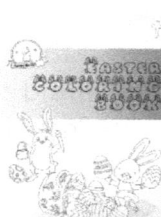

Visit Aryla Publishing website
to sign up for new release books
and free promotions

www.ingramcontent.com/pod-product-compliance
Lightning Source LLC
Chambersburg PA
CBHW071757200326
41520CB00013BA/3291